EARLY PREGNANCY SYMPTOMS

GENERAL GUIDE FOR THE EXPECTING

MOTHER

DR. J. SIMON

Contents

INTRODUCTION

The physical and psychological changes a woman experiences in the first few weeks of her pregnancy, usually prior to missing her period, are known as early pregnancy symptoms. These symptoms are often brought on by hormonal changes that occur when the body adjusts to the presence of a developing embryo. The symptoms of each woman may vary, however these are common early warning signs of pregnancy:

Not Present: One of the most typical early indicators of pregnancy is missing your monthly cycle. This is often when women begin to suspect that they may be pregnant.

Nausea with morning sickness: Nausea is a typical symptom of early pregnancy and is often followed by vomiting. Despite the name "morning sickness," it does not necessarily occur in the morning.

Changes Made to the Breasts: Breast alterations typically occur in the early stages of pregnancy. This may entail breast pain, edema, and darkening of the areolas.

Tired: Being too fatigued or exhausted is a typical symptom. Hormonal fluctuations and increased metabolic demands can contribute to fatigue.

Frequent urination: Hormonal changes in early pregnancy might result in increased blood flow to the kidneys and increased frequency of urination. Increased Odor Perception: Certain women may grow insensitive to certain scents or acquire an allergy to particular fragrances.

Cravings or Aversions to Food: Changes in taste and scent might cause aversions to some foods or urges for others.

Mood Variations: Hormonal fluctuations can impact mood and lead to emotional changes such as irritability, mood swings, or increased feelings.

cramping in the stomach: Mild pains may occur when the uterus begins to expand in order to accommodate the developing embryo.

Changes in Basal Body Temperature: Pregnancy may be indicated by a consistent rise in basal body temperature, which some women track. hemorrhaging during surgery: Some women may experience slight spotting or implantation bleeding around the time of implantation; this could be mistaken for a light phase.

It's important to keep in mind that not all women may have all of these symptoms, and that they can vary in severity. Moreover, many of these symptoms have ties to other medical conditions. A pregnancy suspect can be confirmed with a home pregnancy test or a visit to a healthcare provider.

Understanding the signs of early pregnancy can help people recognize physical changes and take appropriate action, such as getting prenatal care, changing lifestyle choices, and preparing for the journey of conception and delivery.

CHAPTER ONE

Recognizing Early Pregnancy Signs

Recognizing early pregnancy signs is crucial for several reasons, some of which are as follows:

Confirm Pregnancy: Early pregnancy signs, such as breast changes, nausea, and irregular periods, can be used to diagnose pregnancy. Individuals who experience these symptoms are more likely to ask a doctor for confirmation or to obtain a pregnancy test.

Look for Pregnancy Care: Early pregnancy discoveries increase the likelihood that a woman will begin prenatal care straight away. Prenatal care is necessary to monitor the health of the developing fetus and the mother, manage potential risks, and ensure a healthy pregnancy.

Change Your Lifestyle: Those who are aware of the early signs of pregnancy can adjust their lifestyle as necessary. This may mean beginning a healthier diet, avoiding certain drugs and alcohol, and taking prenatal vitamins consistently.

Mental Preparation: Early diagnosis of pregnancy symptoms allows for emotional planning. People are able to process the information, discuss their feelings, and create plans for the upcoming changes in their lives as a result. Couples benefit from it as well. Address Health Concerns: Pregnancy may be impacted in certain women who are taking medication or who already have health problems. When people notice the early indicators of pregnancy, they should consult a doctor to address any potential health problems and, if needed, adjust their medication.

Manage Symptoms: Knowing the warning signs of early pregnancy helps women manage their discomfort and get rid of symptoms like nausea, tiredness, and aching breasts. This could contribute to a more comfortable pregnancy experience.

Financial Administration: When people are aware that a pregnancy is occurring, they can make financial plans. This entails budgeting for future lifestyle adjustments, prenatal care, and childbirth costs.

When to Perform Prenatal Examinations: Early pregnancy detection is necessary for timely prenatal testing and screenings. Certain tests are more effective when performed at specific stages of pregnancy, such as genetic screenings and ultrasounds.

Prepare for labor and delivery: When people are aware of the early indicators of pregnancy, they have more time to educate themselves about labor and delivery, pregnancy, and labor. One may feel more empowered and prepared for the experience of giving birth after reading this information.

Reduce Your Contact with Hazardous Substances: Women who are aware that they are expecting take steps to reduce their exposure to substances that could be harmful to the developing fetus, such as chemicals, medications, and environmental toxins.

Establish a Network of Support: People can notify their support system friends, family, and partners when they become aware of an issue early on. As a result, during the course of the pregnancy, a network of practical and emotional support is formed. In conclusion, recognizing early pregnancy symptoms is one of the most crucial steps to ensuring a safe and well-supported pregnancy.

It makes early medical interventions, lifestyle changes, and mental preparation easier, all of which ultimately lead to better health outcomes for the mother and the growing child.

Common Indices of Early Pregnancy

Women may encounter one or more of the usual early pregnancy symptoms, or they may experience them all at once. It's important to keep in mind that these symptoms can also be associated with other conditions, so it's advisable to confirm your pregnancy by taking a test or consulting a physician.

Common indications of an early pregnancy consist of:

Not Present: Absence of menstrual cycles is often one of the early signs of pregnancy. However, some women may experience little spotting or irregular bleeding.

Nausea with morning sickness: Whether or not vomiting happens, nausea is a common symptom in the early stages of pregnancy. It can trigger by certain meals or smells and occur at any time of day.

Changes Made to the Breasts: Breast modifications, such as discomfort, enlargement, and darkening of the areolas, are common. The breasts may become more sensitive.

Tired: Weariness or excessive fatigue is a common early pregnancy symptom. Hormonal changes and increased metabolic demands both contribute to this fatigue.

Frequent urination: An increased blood flow to the kidneys could result in more urination. This symptom may start early in the pregnancy and continue the entire time.

Increased Odor Perception: Certain women could be more sensitive to scents than others, and certain scents might make you feel queasy or aversional.

Cravings or Aversions to Food: Changes in taste and scent might cause aversions to some foods or urges for others. Food tastes can differ.

Mood Variations: Hormonal fluctuations can lead to increased sentiments, irritability, and mood swings. cramping in the stomach: Mild stomach cramps may occur when the uterus begins to expand to make room for the developing embryo.

Changes in Basal Body Temperature: Pregnancy may be indicated by a consistent rise in basal body temperature, which some women track.

hemorrhaging during surgery: About the time of implantation, some women may have mild spotting or implantation hemorrhage. It is usually lighter than a normal period.

Headaches: Hormonal changes could be the cause of headaches in the early stages of pregnancy.

Some women may experience more intense or frequent feelings.

Feeling faint or lightheaded: Increased blood flow and changes in blood pressure can cause dizziness or lightheadedness.

Constipation: Hormonal changes that affect digestion can cause constipation in some pregnant women.

Enhanced Odor Perception: Some women may have an increased sense of smell in the early stages of pregnancy, which can aggravate aversions or nausea. It's important to remember that these symptoms do not prove or disprove pregnancy.

Using a home pregnancy test or visiting a doctor are the most reliable ways to find out if you are pregnant.

Women can also experience a wide range of symptoms, not all of which will be felt by them in the same way or to the same extent.

Decreased Indications of Early Pregnancy

Even though the typical early pregnancy symptoms are well known, some women may also experience less common symptoms during this time. Individual differences may exist in these symptoms, and women may not always experience them. It's important to keep in mind that these symptoms could also be connected to other illnesses, so it's advisable to confirm the diagnosis by getting tested for pregnancy or seeing a doctor. Some less common early pregnancy symptoms are as follows: Metal taste: A peculiar or metallic aftertaste may be experienced by certain women. This taste experience, often described as bitter or metallic in flavor, may be linked to hormonal changes.

Excessive salivation, or hypersalivation: Early in their pregnancies, some women may experience increased salivation as a result of increased saliva production.

Nasal congestion or hemorrhage: Hormone changes can affect mucous membranes, causing nasal congestion or occasional nosebleeds. Skin Alterations: Some women may experience changes in their skin tone or breakouts of acne. Hormone fluctuations can impact the appearance of the skin.

Skin Discoloration (Chloasma): Chloasma, or skin darkening, is a condition that can affect the face, particularly the cheeks, nose, and forehead. This is sometimes referred to as the "mask of pregnancy." unusually intense thirst some expectant mothers might feel more thirsty than usual. Changes in hormone levels and an increase in blood volume can both contribute to this feeling.

Increased Vaginal Clearance: Changes in cervical mucus production in certain pregnant women may result in an increase in vaginal discharge.

Increased heart rate: Certain women may feel an increase in heart rate in the early stages of pregnancy. This is brought on by modifications to cardiovascular function and an increase in blood volume.

CHAPTER TWO

Variations in Libido: Changes in hormone levels can have an effect on libido, making some women feel more or less attracted to men sexually.

Alterations in the digestive system: Less frequently occurring gastrointestinal symptoms include gas, bloating, and changes in bowel habits. Hormonal changes may have an impact on digestion.

Joint Pain: Certain pregnant women may feel pain or discomfort in their joints, possibly due to changes in the musculoskeletal system.

Headaches: In the early stages of pregnancy, some women may experience migraines despite headaches being a common complaint; this could be due to hormonal changes.

Improved Sensation of Taste: Similar to an enhanced sense of smell, some women may experience changes in taste perception, with some tastes being stronger or more pronounced than others.

Back ache: Certain pregnant women may experience backaches as a result of hormonal fluctuations and their growing uterus.

Palpitations: Some women may experience palpitations or feel as though their hearts are beating too quickly during the first trimester of pregnancy.

It's important to remember that each woman experiences things differently, and not all of them will exhibit these less common symptoms. If there are concerns or doubts about a potential pregnancy, it is recommended to take a pregnancy test and consult with a healthcare provider to get the information you need.

Factors Influencing Symptom Presence and Intensity

Several factors can affect the presence and intensity of early pregnancy symptoms. Pregnant women may perceive their symptoms in a variety of ways because these variables can vary from person to person.

A few of the essential components are:

Hormone Variations: Hormonal imbalances are the main cause of early pregnancy symptoms. Women may have different levels of hormones, such as progesterone, estrogen, and human chorionic gonadotropin (hCG), which can affect when and how severe symptoms appear.

Individual Sensitivity: Every woman's body responds differently to hormonal fluctuations. Some women may experience fewer or milder symptoms, but others may be more sensitive to these shifts and experience more intense symptoms.

Overall Health and Well-Being: The general health and well-being of a woman may have an impact on how she feels during the early stages of her pregnancy. Several factors are involved, such as nutritional status, general health, and previous medical conditions.

Genetic Components: Genetic factors may influence individual differences in how pregnancy symptoms manifest. Genetic variations may affect how the body responds to hormones and adjusts to pregnancy.

Previous Experience with Pregnancy: Women who are pregnant and have given birth before may exhibit different symptoms in their next pregnancy. Pregnancy to pregnancy can cause variations in the body's response to hormonal shifts.

Levels of Stress: Stress levels and mental health conditions may have an impact on how severe pregnancy symptoms are. High levels of stress may exacerbate certain symptoms, but being at ease and relaxed may help the process go more smoothly.

Basic Health Conditions: Diabetes or thyroid problems are two examples of pre-existing medical conditions that may affect a woman's experience of early pregnancy symptoms. It is imperative that these illnesses receive the appropriate medical care.

Drugs and dietary supplements: The effects of some medications or supplements may affect the symptoms. Women who take drugs or supplements may experience changes in how their symptoms present.

Age: The severity of the symptoms could vary depending on age. Pregnancy symptoms may manifest differently in younger and older women due to age-related hormonal changes.

Body Mass Index, or BMI: Body weight and BMI can affect hormonal balance. Depending on their BMI, women may experience variations in the severity of their symptoms. Number of Fetuses: Having multiple fetuses (twins, triplets, etc.) may result in higher hormone levels, which can aggravate symptoms like nausea and breast pain.

Diet and Nutrition: A woman's general health and the nutrients she eats can have an impact on her pregnancy symptoms. Maintaining a healthy diet is crucial when expecting.

State of Hydration: Dehydration can aggravate certain symptoms, such as headaches and vertigo. Maintaining a healthy weight while pregnant requires drinking enough water. It is important to recognize that every pregnancy is unique and that each person's experience with the symptoms of early pregnancy is influenced by the combination of these factors. In order to get guidance and support throughout their pregnancy, it is advised that women talk to their healthcare providers about their symptoms.

Differentiating Pregnancy Symptoms from Other Disorders

Sometimes it's hard to tell pregnancy symptoms apart from other illnesses because some of them are nebulous and can coexist with multiple medical conditions. However, a few factors might make it simpler to distinguish symptoms of pregnancy from those of other illnesses:

The Menstrual Cycle's History: A common sign of early pregnancy is not getting your period. A sexually active woman may consider taking a pregnancy test if she misses her period.

Timing and Pattern of Symptoms: Pregnancy symptoms are often caused by hormonal changes. For example, breast pain and morning sickness may worsen. Observing the timing and pattern of symptoms can provide clues.

Length and Regularity: Pregnancy symptoms frequently persist and intensify with time. Long-lasting, consistent symptoms may be a sign of pregnancy. On the other hand, sporadic or transient symptoms may indicate the presence of other diseases.

Proof via Pregnancy Test: The most accurate way to determine whether someone is pregnant is to use a pregnancy test, either performed by a doctor or at home. Several assays are used to detect the hormone known as human chorionic gonadotropin (hCG), which is released during pregnancy. Specifically, signs Pregnancy is more specifically indicated by some symptoms, such as areolar darkening, implantation bleeding, or particular food cravings. It can be simpler to distinguish pregnancy from other illnesses by being aware of these specific symptoms. Medical Evaluation If symptoms are not clear or if pregnancy is suspected, it is best to get medical attention. Exams and tests may be conducted by medical professionals to determine the cause of symptoms.

Basic Health Conditions: Women with underlying medical conditions can also experience symptoms similar to pregnancy. Disorders such as polycystic ovarian syndrome

(PCOS) are among those that may cause irregular menstrual cycles.

Side effects from medication: Some medications can cause symptoms that mimic those of pregnancy. Reviewing the side effects of any drugs being taken can be educational.

Stressors and Lifestyle: Stress, changes in lifestyle, or significant life events can all aggravate symptoms such as fatigue, appetite swings, and mood swings. An assessment of recent life changes can offer context.

How to Tell PMS from Pregnancy

Sometimes, premenstrual syndrome (PMS) symptoms can be mistaken for early pregnancy symptoms. The key lies in observing how symptoms align with the menstrual cycle.

Pain or discomfort in the pelvis: Pelvic pain or discomfort can be brought on by a variety of conditions, including ovarian cysts and pelvic inflammatory disease (PID).

To determine the cause, a medical professional can conduct assessments. Being mindful of the fact that individual experiences can vary is necessary when approaching the differentiation of symptoms. If there is any uncertainty or concern about a potential pregnancy, it is recommended to seek advice from a healthcare professional to ensure appropriate testing and treatment.

When a pregnancy test is taken can have a significant impact on its accuracy.

The guidelines for when to get a pregnancy test are as follows:

Not Present: The most frequent reason to get a pregnancy test is missed menstruation. If your menstruation is delayed, it is a good idea to get tested. However, some tests are sensitive enough to detect pregnancy even a few days before the menstrual cycle disappears.

Early Pregnancy Testing: A few at-home pregnancy tests are designed to detect pregnancy prior to the absence of menstruation. These tests can provide accurate results several days ahead of your expected period and are typically more sensitive. They might be sold as "early detection tests" or "early pregnancy tests."

Make Use of Your Initial Morning Urine: Pregnancy tests should ideally be taken early in the morning and the first urine used.

This is due to the fact that hCG, or human chorionic gonadotropin, the pregnancy hormone, is easier to find in the morning when its levels are usually higher.

Pay attention to the test guidelines: Follow the instructions on the pregnancy test kit at all times. Each kit may include detailed instructions on when and how to perform the test. When used improperly, the accuracy of the test may suffer.

Comparing Cycles: Regular and Irregular In general, irregularly cyclical women can use the lack of a period as a signal to get tested.

Those with irregular cycles may find it more difficult to predict when to get tested, and other symptoms or factors may need to be taken into account.

hemorrhaging during surgery: If you experience mild spotting, also known as implantation bleeding, at the time of implantation, you might choose to wait a few days to get a pregnancy test.

Days seven to ten after ovulation: If you are tracking ovulation and know when you ovulated, waiting seven to ten days after ovulation before taking a test can increase the accuracy of the results. Comparing Digital and Line Tests Digital pregnancy tests may display the words "pregnant" or "not pregnant" clearly, while line tests may display lines that vary in intensity. You could choose digital exams if you want results that are clear.

Check Again if the Answer Is No: If the test is negative but you still suspect pregnancy, you can choose to retest a few days later or wait until your period is more obviously overdue. Remember that while home pregnancy tests, when used properly, can provide very accurate results, they are not perfect.

If you have any doubts or get contradicting results, you should see a healthcare provider for further evaluation or a blood test. In addition, maintaining a healthy lifestyle and taking prenatal vitamins are advised for those who are trying to conceive or who suspect they may be pregnant.

Coping Strategies and Self-Repair

Pregnant women can better handle the emotional and physical changes that come with their pregnancy by creating self-care routines that prioritize their physical and mental health.

Here are some self-care tips and coping strategies related to pregnancy:

Optimal Eating Practices: Maintain a healthy, well-balanced diet to support both your own health and the growth of the unborn child. Ascertain that you are getting enough calcium, iron, folic acid, and omega-3 fatty acids, among other essential nutrients. consuming lots of water Drink plenty of water throughout the day to ensure that you are properly hydrated. Constipation symptoms can be alleviated and overall health is enhanced by consuming adequate water.

Regular Exercise: Observe your physician's recommendations and engage in regular, moderate exercise. Pregnant yoga, low-impact aerobics, walking, and swimming can all help maintain physical fitness while boosting mood and reducing stress.

Adequate Rest and Sleep: Prioritize getting enough rest and sleep. Pregnancy can involve a lot of physical demands, so it's critical for general health and vitality to get enough sleep.

Managing Stress: Take part in stress-relieving exercises such as pregnancy yoga, deep breathing, mindfulness, and meditation. Stress management is essential for both your own health and the health of the unborn child.

Regular Prenatal Care: Observe your doctor's advice and don't miss any of your prenatal appointments. Regular check-ups help monitor both your and the unborn child's health.

Discover for Yourself: Enroll in birthing and parenting classes to learn about the various stages of pregnancy, labor, and postpartum care.

Acquiring knowledge can lessen anxiety and increase confidence.

Establish a Relationship: Establish relationships with loved ones, friends, and other expectant mothers to build a support system.

Discuss your experiences, concerns, and joys with people who can relate to you and offer support.

Take Care of Yourself: Allow yourself some time to relax and enjoy. It's imperative to look after oneself during pregnancy, whether that means getting a massage, taking a warm bath, or just spending time by oneself.

Express Your Feelings: Discuss your feelings with your friends, your significant other, or a mental health professional. During a pregnancy, a range of emotions may surface, so open communication is essential. Having a positive body image Recognize and accept the changes your body is going through. Respect the experience of pregnancy and highlight its benefits. Consider scheduling massages or maternity photo shoots as ways to savor the moment.

Aromatherapy: Use aromatherapy with calming fragrances to promote relaxation. Essential oils that promote calmness, like chamomile or lavender, can be used appropriately.

CHAPTER THREE

Wear-anywhere clothing: Invest in comfortable, breathable maternity clothing. Well-fitting clothing can reduce discomfort and boost confidence.

Pelvic Floor Exercises: Exercise your pelvic floor to strengthen the muscles that support your pelvic organs. Kegel exercises are beneficial before, during, and after childbirth.

Plan Your Repose After Giving Birth: Make time for rest and recovery after giving birth. After giving birth, arrange for a calm and supportive environment and make plans for help from family or friends.

Keep in mind that every pregnancy is unique, so your self-care routine should be tailored to your own needs. Consult your healthcare provider before making any significant changes to your diet, exercise routine, or self-care routine while you're pregnant.

Lifestyle Changes during the Early Pregnancy

During the first trimester of pregnancy, lifestyle changes are essential to support the health of both the mother and the fetus. The following are some significant lifestyle adjustments to consider:

Optimal Eating Practices: Have a nutrient-dense, well-balanced diet that includes lots of fruits, vegetables, whole grains, lean meats, dairy products, and dairy alternatives. Verify that you are getting all the nutrients you need, including folic acid, calcium, iron, and omega-3 fatty acids. consuming lots of water To stay properly hydrated throughout the day, sip on plenty of water. Adequate hydration not only improves overall health but also mitigates the symptoms of common pregnancy ailments like constipation.

Avoid Harmful Substances: Give up alcohol, cigarettes, and recreational drug use. These medications may cause problems and have negative effects on the development of the embryo. Don't drink too much coffee. Reduce your intake of caffeinated drinks. High coffee consumption has been associated with an increased risk of miscarriage. Find out from your doctor how much caffeine is suitable for you to take.

Regular Exercise: Regularly engage in moderate exercise as directed by your healthcare provider. Exercises like swimming, walking, and prenatal yoga help enhance overall health and physical fitness.

Enough Sleep: Prioritize getting enough rest and sleep. Pregnancy can be physically demanding, and getting enough sleep is essential for the health of the expectant mother as well as the development of the growing child.

Manage Your Tension: Employ techniques for reducing stress, such as deep breathing, mindfulness, and meditation. Chronic stress during pregnancy may have negative effects on both the mother and the fetus.

Pregnancy-related vitamins: Take prenatal vitamins as directed by your physician. You can be sure that you are getting essential nutrients from these supplements, like folic acid, which is critical for the development of the fetal neural tube.

Avoid putting the environment at risk: Minimize your exposure to environmental hazards such as pollution, radiation, and hazardous compounds. Verify whether working is safe for you during pregnancy, and discuss any concerns you may have with your healthcare provider. Regular

Checkups on Mothers: Attend all of your prenatal appointments on time. Regular visits allow your doctor to monitor your fetus's growth, keep an eye on your health, and address any problems that may arise.

Discover for Yourself: Enroll in birthing and parenting classes to learn about the various stages of pregnancy, labor, and postpartum care. Having information reduces anxiety and enables you to make informed decisions.

Maintain an Appropriate Weight: Aim for a healthy weight gain during pregnancy as losing or gaining too much weight could be harmful. Consult your physician about appropriate weight goals.

Pelvic Floor Exercises: Do pelvic floor exercises, or Kegels, to strengthen the muscles that support the pelvic organs. These can be beneficial throughout the pregnancy and after giving birth. Keep Up Adequate Hygiene: To stay healthy, practice good hygiene. When taking care of yourself, wash your hands often, handle food carefully, and practice good hygiene.

Engaging with the Healthcare Professional: Maintain open channels of communication with your healthcare provider. Discuss any concerns, changes in symptoms, or intended lifestyle adjustments you have for the impending pregnancy.

It's crucial to tailor lifestyle adjustments to your particular needs and seek guidance from your healthcare provider. Since each pregnancy is unique, getting personalized care is crucial to having a positive pregnancy experience.

CONCLUSION

The process of becoming pregnant drastically alters a person's body, emotions, and way of life. From the first signs of conception to the end of childbirth, the process is characterized by joy, excitement, and the nurturing of new life. An expectant mother's body undergoes amazing changes to support her developing child, and she must manage a range of emotions, from excitement to vulnerable times. Pregnancy is full of exciting experiences, like your first ultrasound, feeling the baby move, and finally holding your little one in your arms. Throughout this journey, it is crucial for the mother and developing child to maintain their health through self-care, good nutrition, and prenatal care. Changing one's lifestyle to incorporate stress reduction, a balanced diet, and frequent exercise can all contribute to a happy and healthy pregnancy. Consulting with medical professionals, attending prenatal checkups, and seeking guidance on various pregnancy-related matters are all parts of a well-supported journey. A vital support system can be provided by family, friends, or other loved ones in the form of both practical and emotional assistance. The birth of a precious child and the beginning of the postpartum period coincide with the end of a pregnancy. Pregnancy strengthens the bond between mother and child as she embraces the challenges and joys of parenting and spends quality time attending to her child's needs and watching them develop.

The pregnancy journey comes to an end with the child's birth, but the profound effects endure a lifetime. Memories of those first flutters, the excitement of ultrasounds, and the wonder of creating new life are all woven throughout the experience of being a parent.

Even as the family grows and changes, the memories of the pregnant journey are a treasured part of their overall story, which is one of love, resiliency, and the beginning of a new chapter in life.

THE END

www.ingramcontent.com/pod-product-compliance
Lightning Source LLC
Chambersburg PA
CBHW060845260726
48661CB00002B/618